Flourishing Healthcare Professionals

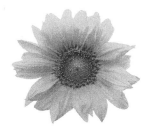

LOUISE BRODA

2QT (Publishing) Ltd

First Edition published 2015 by

2QT Limited (Publishing)
Unit 5 Commercial Courtyard
Duke Street
Settle
North Yorkshire
BD24 9RH

Copyright © Louise Broda
The right of Louise Broda to be identified as the author
of this work has been asserted by her in accordance
with the Copyright, Designs and Patents Act 1988

All rights reserved. This book is sold subject to the
condition that no part of this book is to be reproduced,
in any shape or form. Or by way of trade, stored in a
retrieval system or transmitted in any form or by any
means, electronic, mechanical, photocopying, recording,
be lent, re-sold, hired out or otherwise circulated in any
form of binding or cover other than that in which it is
published and without a similar condition, including this
condition being imposed on the subsequent purchaser,
without prior permission of the copyright holder.

Illustrations by: Emily Yearsley
Cover images: Shutterstock.com

Printed by Lighting Source UK

A CIP catalogue record for this book is
available from the British Library

ISBN 978-1-910077-38-2

Acknowledgements

A special thank you to Salmaan Sana, Georgie Oldfield, Gordon Turnbull, Doug Newburg, Rick Hanson and Andy Kemp who have all inspired me and given up their time to be interviewed. Without their generous offerings this would have been a very different book.

I am also very grateful for all the help and support from Catherine Cousins, Karen Holmes and Hilary Pitt in helping my vision come to print. Their fine tuning of this manuscript and their belief in me is greatly appreciated.

About the author

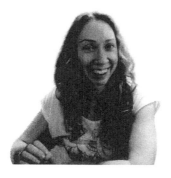

I am a physiotherapist by training though my keen interest in the mind-body link has led me to an MSc in Sport Psychology and training in Neurolinguistic Programming (NLP).

After personal experience of empathy fatigue, I learned the importance of self-awareness and self-care. I am now passionate about the wellbeing of healthcare professionals and helping them to recognise that they are the most important person in their work.

Introduction

*'The true way to render ourselves happy is to
love our work and find in it our pleasure.'*

Francoise de Motteville

THE IMPORTANCE OF compassion in healthcare is a hot topic and frequently in the news of late. I am a strong advocate for compassion and its crucial role in maintaining a caring relationship with patients. However, I am here to defend the hundreds, if not thousands, of healthcare professionals who were always compassionate, until the nature of their work and lack of self-care adversely affected them.

I am passionate about the care of healthcare professionals and helping you recognise that you are the most important person in your work. We are taught that we must empathise with and be compassionate towards our patients. We forget (or were never taught) that first we must be compassionate towards ourselves.

You may not be able to change the healthcare system but you can influence how you exist in it and react to it… I want you to thrive rather than just survive! I want to inspire and make a difference by giving others what I wish I had learned at university. I also want to ensure that good healthcare practitioners stop leaving the profession because they feel they are not good enough or because they are exhausted. There is a different way!

As well as a lot of my colleagues, I feel disheartened and upset by some of the recent press coverage about hospital scandals and standards of care. Much of it has been very negative and it is frustrating to read when I know that there are incredibly good levels of care being offered all over the country and the world. However, I understand the reason that levels of compassion – and thus care – can decline.

The focus now is on ensuring that we train compassionate healthcare professionals. I agree that this is imperative – but I am aware that there are hundreds of professionals who were excited, passionate and caring when they started their careers but are now exhausted. They were never taught how to protect themselves in the caring relationship. They have either become slightly dissociated by building up a protective mental barrier in order to cope, or more worryingly, have left the profession altogether in favour of a less exhausting career.

I want to show an alternative approach by offering a book that recognises that these people have not failed; they were not taught to use the right tools in the first place. I want to show you there is a way back to being the caring and compassionate healthcare professional you always wanted to be. I also want to cultivate resilient students and encourage them to flourish!

Since I started writing a blog two years ago, I have discovered a passion for writing in a very honest and open way. I believe that we should not be constrained by convention, and feel privileged to live in a time where I can challenge accepted norms. I have had to be brave and expose my vulnerabilities as I wrote this book because it is something that I feel deeply passionate about; I could easily have written a less personal book that did not speak from the heart but may have been more acceptable to the medical world. That didn't feel right to me and I would not have been true to myself if I had taken that approach. To appease those of you with a need for a more traditional research-based approach, there is a wealth of factual information in the resource section (in addition to a large practical skills section, Chapter 8).

It is amazing to follow your passions but even when you do, you come across obstacles that test and frustrate you and at times make you feel like giving up. These are the real tests. Even though writing this book has been a largely enjoyable process for me, it has tested me and I have learned a lot. I had a period where I was really stuck with writing and, after realising that I hadn't done any exercise for a while, got stuck into a workout. It made a massive difference because it helped me to remember what I loved and how I wanted to feel.

I want to share with you tips from people I admire, who have inspired me and from whom I have learned a huge amount about health and wellbeing. I hope that by helping you understand a little more about how your mind and body work (and the interplay between them) you can become less stressed and more relaxed, and remember what it is like to feel really well. This includes allowing yourself time to play and enjoy your passions!

Key messages:

- You can regain your passion for your job.
- You need to care for yourself *before* you can care for others.
- Compassion is good for your health.
- Remember why you went into the healthcare professions in the first place.
- You are human and therefore you will face stress and upset. This is normal; you don't have to be superhuman to be a healthcare professional. Your needs are important too!

'Don't ever lose sight of the gift that is you. When life seems to knock you down, get back up and get back in the game. 'Remember what you're made of. Remember what's flowing in your veins. Remember what you were given, and remember what you went out and created on your own. Like any great masterpiece, you're not done yet. Inside you is the best of everyone who has come before you – and the best of everyone yet to be. You can forget some of what life hands you, but never forget who you are. You are a gift to the world!'

Rachel Snyder

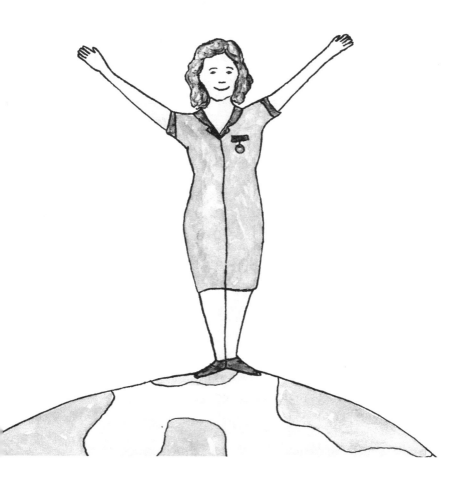

My story

'If you are attached to being the lover or the giver – as opposed to giving when giving is needed or loving when loving is needed – then you are bound to be depleted. I must always maintain my own care or I have nothing to give from (periodically, it is appropriate to take a break from giving).'

Reverend Amy Wiggins

Compassion for my fatigue

I THINK I am nosey at heart. I love people and love finding out about what makes them tick. From a young age I was always good at listening and this was my default setting rather than talking … I would make sure I got in first to ask how the other person was. I was never taught that my listening skills, which are so valuable when working with people, could actually make me ill!

I was attracted to physiotherapy as a career after school because it felt like the perfect way to combine my love of all the sciences (especially human biology) with my love of sport and my unquenchable thirst for finding out about people. I also had a little extra insight as my mum was a physiotherapist, though if anything she tried to put me off, as she didn't want to feel that she had influenced me in any way. Like many of us who are attracted into the health and caring professions, I worked hard at school; I had perfectionist tendencies and put a lot of pressure on myself to do well.

At university, our compassionate and empathic sides were encouraged and rightly so, as I truly believe that showing you care can be a huge part of the reason why someone gets better. I was never warned that my caring nature could actually damage me.

I experienced many different clinical placements as a student: from respiratory physiotherapy in intensive care; neuro-rehabilitation and care of the elderly, to general injuries in outpatient physiotherapy. I vividly remember spending four weeks on an oncology ward where quite a few of the terminally ill patients died. I didn't understand how I would ever cope with this. My supervisor's only advice was to ask if I wanted to sit in the office for a few minutes before I got on with the rest of the day. I decided that I wasn't cut out for oncology physio and have never worked in that area again.

Because our feelings were not discussed, I believed that I should have been able to cope, and I learned (wrongly, I now know) to keep things to myself. I may never have worked again in this area but I feel strongly that if my supervisor had handled things differently that placement would have been a very different experience. In hindsight, it could have given me greater skills and understanding about how your own emotions can and will affect you.

When I graduated, I enjoyed being taken seriously as a professional. I have always loved to talk to patients about themselves and it felt natural to empathise with their injuries or problems and listen to the person beneath the injury. I used to go home and worry about patients and how I could best help them; even then I knew that this was not healthy, but I cared so much for them and wanted to do my absolute best to help. I had a fantastic supervisor who could see herself in me and encouraged me not to think about patients when I went home but her advice didn't help. I didn't know how to change without losing some of my ability to care.

I really enjoyed my job and felt lucky to be doing something I loved. Then I started getting ill regularly, usually with a cold every six months or so; it would often linger and I would be left with extreme fatigue for weeks. I have always loved exercising and being so exhausted was an inconvenience that frustrated me. Eventually the fatigue would pass and I would throw myself back into working and exercising. I was always busy; I had a fantastic group of friends; I was always looking for further courses, particularly in sports which would help me develop into an even better physiotherapist. I was very driven to improve and learn all I could learn, not just to tick the box to continue my professional development because I had to. At that stage I had no idea that what I really needed was to start caring for myself properly and improve my work-life balance.

As I grew more experienced and changed jobs, I worried less about patients in the evenings. Some would stick in my head overnight but I had less of the all-consuming worry about helping them. Despite this, I still had bouts of extreme fatigue and spells where I felt incredibly resentful of patients and their problems; these uncaring emotions were not like me at all. On more than one occasion these feelings led me to question whether I was really meant to be a physiotherapist.

It was not until I heard about compassion fatigue (or empathy fatigue, as I prefer to call it) and began reading

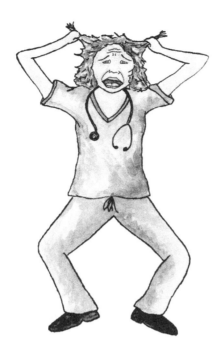

more about it, that I felt like someone truly understood what I had been going through. Looking back, I can identify with so many of the symptoms and the lack of emotional self-care.

Some signs and symptoms of empathy fatigue (this is by no means an exhaustive list):

- Chronically tired/exhausted (physically or emotionally)
- Feelings of helplessness/hopelessness
- Feeling bad or cynical about oneself
- Dulled emotions
- Decreased motivation and drive
- Anger

- Blaming others
- Depression/low mood
- Frequent headaches
- Gastrointestinal complaints
- Overly high expectations
- Hypertension
- Inability to maintain a balance of empathy and objectivity
- Irritable
- Low self-esteem
- Disturbed sleep
- Working too much (Rothschild, 2006)

I have certainly seen a few of these symptoms in myself at one time or another! Do you? Displaying any of these symptoms does not mean that you are uncaring or that you should be doing something different, it may just mean that you are absorbing things from people that you are not aware of and that you need to look after yourself more. I am a firm believer that prevention is always better than cure ... so if you can take my message on board and never get to the point that I did, fantastic!

As health professionals we are expected to be caring but we are often given little or no advice on the importance of self-care and that caring about others can affect our health. It is not something that I was ever taught at university. Now, in retrospect I see that it is something that made me ill on more than one occasion and sapped my energy and enthusiasm for my work for years.

Self-awareness

For me, recovery started with becoming more self-aware.

It is easy to coast through life without much awareness of ourselves and to get stressed and stuck with life. I have done a lot of self-development over the last twelve years and it has been much more important than all the continuing professional development courses I have done. Most of us have to do mandatory training annually on topics such as basic life support – but we don't see ourselves as so important. Should we be doing annual self-development courses?

Self-awareness and personal development are themes that I have come across in my own life and are persistent threads in this book. They should be ongoing, evolving processes that are encouraged at university and in the world of work. It is not always an easy process but it teaches us a lot.

Through my years of wondering if I was cut out to be a physio or if I would be better doing something else, I have done three key courses. These courses led me to some amazing people (some of whom are in this book) and were significant personal milestones. They gave me a broad range of skills and knowledge that I added to my professional portfolio – and they gave me so much more.

The first course was in Neurolinguistic Programming (NLP) for sport. From this I rediscovered my love of the sporting world, becoming more interested in the brain and psychology, as well as learning a lot about myself. Afterwards I was still frustrated with physio and chose to complete an MSc in Sport Psychology. I loved this and felt that I had found my new direction. The positive world of working with sport and understanding psychology on a deeper level hooked me, though I couldn't get rid of my physio roots and kept finding that I was relating back to my experience as a physio. One of the insights I discovered on this course was that my frustrations were borne out of the 'Medical Model' training and approach we follow as healthcare professionals. I had a *eureka* moment when I realised that it was this way of looking at patients and disease which felt so restrictive. I had always felt that health and wellbeing were much broader topics than the way we generally look at health in the western world (much more on this later!).

After finishing my MSc I needed a rest; it had been an exhausting year and there was a lot of stress in my personal life. I chose to do some locum work and accidentally fell into working for the military. I was very lucky to be able to introduce some of my newfound sport psychology skills such as goal setting and relaxation into the rehab environment. I also began to realise that I didn't want to start at the bottom of the ladder again as a sport psychologist. Maybe I needed to combine my skills in a different environment?

The military was quite different to the National Health Service (NHS) and possibly more similar to my experience of working in private hospitals, particularly because of the resources available. However, it threw up its own challenges since a lot more of the patients had more obvious (to me at least) psychological issues.

I have always believed that the mind and body are connected and that we don't get our treatment right when we only address one aspect. By chance, I read a short article in *Frontline* (the UK's monthly physio magazine) by Georgie Oldfield who seemed to be speaking my language! One thing led to another and I completed the SIRPA (Stress Illness Recovery Practitioners Association) Practitioner course which confirmed my belief that the mind-body connection is complex, fascinating and underestimated. I went into each course thinking that it would give me skills that would help my patients; they have, because they have helped me learn so much about myself. You have to be open to such courses and to be vulnerable; if you are, you will get so much back in return.

It's one thing to start becoming self-aware; next we need to make use of this knowledge and do something with it.

Choosing to be kind to ourselves

Compassion is not a luxury; it is a necessity for our patients and, more importantly, our own wellbeing. We can't truly practice compassion towards others if we can't treat ourselves kindly.

In our training we are taught that we must be objective but from this objective stance you cannot access your compassionate side. Not only will this approach make connecting with the patient much harder, it can also make you more susceptible to empathy fatigue, burnout or exhaustion. It can disconnect us from the true reason why we do what we do and why we went into healthcare in the first place.

'I found that the biggest reason people aren't more self-compassionate is that they are afraid they'll become self-indulgent. They believe self-criticism is what keeps them in line. Most people have gotten it wrong because our culture says being hard on yourself is the way to be.'

Dr Kristen Neff

The guru of self-compassion, Kristen Neff, has written and talked extensively on this topic. There are copious amounts of research demonstrating that self-compassion promotes self-improvement, decreases comparisons to others, can protect against anxiety and promote psychological resilience (see the resource section). Learning to become more self-compassionate is a vital component of our growth as health professionals and should be integral to our education and practice. When we are kind to ourselves, we tend to project more warmth and understanding to our patients. Our increased kindness towards ourselves helps to temper our judgments about ourselves and others.

We are taught from a young age to work hard, strive to be better and be the best we can be. I agree that we are all here to be the best versions of ourselves ... but sometimes I feel that instead of the inner critic pushing us to work harder and strive for more, it does the opposite and we get in our own way (see Chapter 8 for a range of practical tools to help).

I was the good girl at school and enjoyed it. I strived to get good grades but along the way I was incredibly harsh on myself. I told myself off when I felt that I had done a less than perfect job – and I still have to keep this side of me in check if I am stressed.

At work, I always remembered the one patient who frustrated me because I couldn't work out what was going on with them and why they were not getting better, rather than the many with whom I succeeded.

I failed my driving test twice before I passed and felt like a failure. I wasn't used to failing and I wasn't used to speaking to myself kindly and compassionately at such times. I was harsh on myself when I failed a couple of assignments during my MSc; realistically I was trying to be superwoman and do too much, studying a topic that was different to my job – but I had never failed like that before.

I have begun to realise that it is a choice: we can keep being harsh and criticising ourselves for not doing a perfect job (whatever that is!) or choose to allow the compassion we have for others to shine over ourselves. Life is not always what you want it to be; you cannot control everything and being self-critical only makes life harder.

When you start to realise that *you* are the most important person and what you feel and think about yourself not only matters a great deal, but is also projected to others, it makes you think. Being kind to yourself (especially in moments where you feel like you have failed) is essential and it gives you a chance to change things. It does not mean turning a blind eye to something you could have done better but it is an opportunity to grow.

If you find this thought difficult to accept, how would you react if your best friend was overwhelmed by a tough situation? Would you criticise them or would you offer kind and supportive words?

Be kind to yourself!

Caring for yourself and putting yourself first

'You can't do anything well or for the long term without loving yourself first. When you love yourself, you care about your body, and you care about what you put into it. You also care about the thoughts you choose to think.'

Louise Hay

How important is being caring in your job? Do you think that patients would get better if you didn't care and ignored how they felt, or if you didn't want to listen to their feelings? We probably all agree that caring for our patients is important and that we need to come across as caring professionals. It is arguable that this is, in fact, *the* most important factor in our work.

Knowing that someone cares can instantly make you feel better but do we apply the same rule in caring for ourselves? Working in the health professions, we are often very empathic to everyone *except* the one person who matters the most ... ourselves.

Ask yourself:
- What do I do to care for myself?
- What do I do to reward myself?
- How often do I take time to nurture myself?
- What *could* I do to care for myself more?
- How would caring for myself more make me feel?

My frustration with the lack of recognition of this problem leads me to where I am today. If we work with people a lot, helping or advising in some capacity or just being there for them, we are usually attracted to these jobs because we like people. We often put others' needs before our own and that is often the killer blow to our own health.

Over the years, I have learned a lot about how to go from barely surviving as a healthcare professional to reconnecting with why I went into the profession in the first place. It is not easy and it is an ongoing process. I want to share with you some of the people who have helped and inspired me along the way, in addition to giving you a library of practical tools (Chapter 8) and resources that I hope will help you so that, in turn, you can truly flourish!

The compassion of why we care

*'TIf you want others to be happy, practice compassion.
If you want to be happy, practice compassion.'*

His Holiness the Dalai Lama

I WAS INTRODUCED to Salmaan Sana via a friend. He is a passionate speaker and honest proponent of compassion. Despite being ill as a child and growing up with a dislike of hospitals, he had some amazing experiences which made him want to be a doctor. Following on from working as a carer and a hospital lab assistant, he finally went to medical school.

After becoming a member of the International Federation of Medical Students Association (IFMSA), Salmaan discovered his passion which later took him away from medical school. The IFMSA exists for, and is led by, medical students worldwide; it is a non-government organization within the World Health Organisation. It aims to inspire medical students to develop leadership skills to take on challenges and improve the world around them; hopefully this will enable doctors to become more culturally aware and sensitive physicians.

Feeling his motivation slipping away in the first year of his medical studies, Salmaan questioned why he was starting to lose his passion. After a lot of deliberating, he decided to stop his medical training because he felt he could make more impact in compassionate healthcare or leadership in healthcare. He started his own company and is now involved in projects such as the Healthcare Leadership Summer School, and is the Zero Generation Trainer and Compassion Project Leader at the Medical Center of Leeuwaarden in the Netherlands.

Compassion

'The suffering of others can be met with either empathy or compassion. We have observed that empathically sharing others' pain can increase one's own negative feelings, whereas compassion is associated with having more positive feelings. Importantly, both empathy and compassion can be trained and even short-term training of these social emotions can change the feelings one experiences and the way the brain functions.'

Dr Olga Klimecki.

Compassion is multifaceted and is ultimately about action; even the art of listening is an active demonstration of compassion. Compassion is kind, caring and strives to help others.

Think about it. What does compassion mean to you? What does it feel like for someone to do something compassionate for you, or to have compassion for you?

*'I would rather make mistakes in kindness and compassion
than work miracles in unkindness and hardness.'*

Mother Teresa

Compassion for Care was set up in 2010 by medical students, with the understanding that we should work from a place of compassion – beginning with ourselves. With Salmaan as a core team member, it was started because of personal frustrations and the wish to see change within the healthcare system.

After I came across the topic of compassion fatigue, I started reading about compassion and came across a huge, and constantly growing, bank of resources and research (see the resource section for these). It's funny how:

'When the student is ready, the teacher appears.'

I felt as if these things had been waiting for me to find them! I recall discovering that a one-day workshop on compassion was going to be held in my local area. It felt so right for me to be there – even though I was definitely in the minority as a physiotherapist, with most of the other attendees being counsellors and psychologists. From this I discovered the Compassionate Mind Foundation (and Google group). This has been a brilliant resource where like-minded people share stories and research. It inspired me to read more on the topic of compassion and to see how it can help us become better healthcare professionals, not just for our patients but for ourselves.

I agree with Salmaan that we need to make compassion a part of healthcare education. There is plenty of compassion in healthcare though at present our healthcare systems are very outcome based, measured by efficiency and outcomes, with the human side getting little or no attention. This can be strange and frustrating for both the professionals and for patients. Over the years I have become frustrated with systems and particularly with managers who want to measure everything. Medicine is not just about science; it is also an art. The human aspects cannot be measured by scales and numbers. Most of us who go into healthcare are not thinking about outcomes and efficiency; the energy that drives us in our work comes from within. Compassion for Care was born from this belief.

I appreciate that to a certain extent we need measureable outcomes but I feel that we have become obsessed with them. By having a prescriptive recipe for treating patients, we sideline the other factors that contribute to why someone gets better. We also forget why we, as healthcare professionals, do what we do.

As students and new graduates, we are often science- and fact-based (I know that I was). We want to know what works and we don't have the experience to trust ourselves and listen to what the patient really needs.

'In our training we are taught we must be objective. But from an objective stance, no one has access to his/her human strengths. Objectivity makes healthcare workers vulnerable to burnout. It prevents us from finding meaning.'

Rachel Ramem

Compassion is a way back to the art of what we do as healthcare professionals, the intangible and difficult to measure aspects that are often more important than the aspects we can measure.

It is not always easy to be compassionate though; there are many things that can get in the way of our compassion even when we are trying so very hard to maintain it.

Compassion blocks

Obstacles to compassion:
- Stress
- The system
- Anger
- Perception of not having enough time
- Fear
- Competition

One of the major blocks that surprised me is competition. I am competitive by nature and recently I've discovered just how competitive I can be since I took up stand-up paddle boarding! Imagine a narrow surfboard with the addition of a long paddle and you are pretty close! I have been well and truly bitten by the bug. At the start, I didn't know that you could race in this sport but now I find that racing is fun and definitely fires up my love of a challenge!

Competition can be healthy in sport, and in a lot of areas in life, but I feel that there are some areas where competition is *not* healthy for you or others around you. One of those is in your work as a healthcare professional.

Doctors reading this may be disagreeing – but I'm referring to all health professionals, as well as doctors.

We assume that people who go into the healthcare professions care about others. I am not naïve enough to think that this is an absolute rule, though I am an optimist and believer in people. I do know that, despite the negative press about the lack of compassion and caring in the health professions, most people are compassionate when they start out.

Ultimately my job (along with that of all of my colleagues) is to help my patients and make their life better. By the very nature of the people that we are and what we wish for ourselves, I feel that this should extend to those we work with. However, I have witnessed how these sentiments have been pushed aside and forgotten about.

Why can we be so thoughtful and caring towards our patients but fail to recognise what is going on in a colleague's life? Are we too busy to see it – or do we believe that we should be tough enough not to be affected by the emotions of those around us?

Why do some of us feel the need to compete and be better than our colleagues? Who is to say that one person is right and another is wrong? Surely medicine is about learning and developing. Some of you will argue that medicine is black and white; I would argue that it has many shades of grey that need to be seen and appreciated rather than ignored. It is not a failure to admit that there are things you don't know.

Reminding yourself of the 'why'

In his training and lectures Salmaan often asks: 'Why did you ever start studying or working within the profession? Why do you still do that today?'

These are questions that Robin Youngson talks about in his book *Time to Care*. It seems obvious that we should remember our 'why', but even as students we often lose a grip on this.

'He who knows his why can bear any how.'
Victor Frankle

We all have our own reasons for going into a job, though often as healthcare professionals our reasons are a little stronger; there is something that attracts us towards careers that on the one hand can be so exhausting and on the other are so rewarding.

When I went for an interview at university, the selection day involved lots of practical tasks in addition to a group interview; they specifically avoided asking us why we wanted to be physiotherapists. I left convinced that I had not got in but was elated to discover a few weeks later that I had. It was a great university and I think that the practical side of the interview was brilliant for working out who would make a good physiotherapist. Looking back, however, this process made it easy to lose sight of the reason why I had decided to become a physio. I think that it is important to keep in touch with the passion that drives us towards these professions, not just through university but during our working lives.

Certain patients remind you why you went into the profession in the first place; I had one of those recently. He had had chronic shin pain for years which failed to respond to rehab. He came to the rehab centre for a three-week course which was largely exercise-based, though there was a significant education element. After I delivered a lecture on pain to the group, he commented that he had never thought that some of the stresses in his life could have any impact on his physical symptoms. After talking to him on a one-to-one basis he opened up to me about some of the emotional issues he had been through in the past year and with his consent I was able to refer him to a Chartered Psychiatric

Nurse (CPN) to help. By the end of the three weeks, he was running pain free and described feeling as if a magic wand had been waved. I was proud of this patient for opening up and accepting help and am convinced that it was not just the rehab that allowed him to make such an improvement. I felt rather emotional as he described how he felt but I also felt proud that I had helped him on his journey to recovery. Remember these patients and allow yourself to connect with these moments.

Taking care of yourself during the day

Like all of the inspiring people I interviewed for this book, Salmaan believes that spending time each day taking care of yourself is imperative. I know that this can feel selfish at times, but it is not about spending lots of money or lots of time on yourself. It is exactly the opposite. Taking moments for yourself between patients at the beginning or end of the day is far from selfish because it will help you to give back more.

Ask yourself:
- What can I do during the day to take care of myself?
- What do I need to do to stay healthy?
- What do I need to do in order to engage me with compassion?

Be realistic and understand that there may be some constraints because of your workload, though there is often more wiggle room than you think!

I have compiled an extensive list in the Practical Skills chapter (Chapter 8) that I hope will help with this if you are struggling for ideas. The list is far from exhaustive; once you start to allow yourself to think about the little things, you will come up with many more that will work for you.

Salmaan's top five tips

1. Remember why you started working in healthcare and why you are working in healthcare today.
2. What is it that you need to stay motivated and passionate in your work during the day?
3. How do you make sure you take care of yourself during working shifts?
4. Which small change could you put into action to create a more engaging environment for yourself and your colleagues/patients?
5. How would you want to be treated if you were a patient yourself?

The mind and body are connected!

ONE THING THAT really gets me passionate is how amazing our bodies are! I loved biology at school and was fascinated by the human body (the inner workings of a plant seemed boring to me in comparison). What I find most incredible is the intricate relationship between the mind and the body.

Western medical practice is underpinned by the belief that the mind and body are two separate entities. We generally go to one person to treat our back pain and another person if we need help with our 'minds'. As a physiotherapist I was deeply frustrated by this approach because it did not sit well with what I believed to be true. The medical model is concerned with treating symptoms and making the all-important diagnosis.

I felt like I was speaking a foreign language and so for years I spoke the 'language' of everyone around me as it conformed to what I had been taught and what the majority of Western medicine is based on.

Then I read an article by Georgie Oldfield which felt like it was speaking to that intuitive part of me, acknowledging what I had always felt. Georgie is an inspiring and pioneering physiotherapist who wanted answers to the questions that she was constantly facing with her patients. She began to research and develop her expertise into the Stress Illness Recovery Practitioners Association (SIRPA) www.sirpauk.com.

I completed one of Georgie's courses and found that it addressed many of my own unanswered questions about why certain patients presented with certain conditions, or why they didn't respond to treatment the way I had hoped. It was also (like so many courses, when you are open to them) a journey in self-discovery and self-care. Her work is truly inspiring and it is setting a new trend in the path of healthcare to help us tackle some of the blocks within our patients which prevent them from flourishing ... and more importantly within ourselves.

Recognising the mind-body connection

Georgie is a physiotherapist with more than thirty years' experience who is breaking new ground and making people think. In her early years, she chose to specialise in respiratory care in a large hospital in the UK. After a while she became frustrated with the limitations of physiotherapists and other healthcare professionals in truly dealing with pain. Her frustrations were also borne out of personal experience. She developed severe pain in both thumbs and index fingers without any apparent cause – and as a physiotherapist pain anywhere could be quite debilitating for her. After two sessions of acupuncture, the pain resolved completely. This spurred Georgie on to train in acupuncture. In retrospect, she realised how stressed she was at that point in her life. Her pain resolution also coincided with her seeing a rheumatologist who reassured her that the pain was from osteoarthritis rather than rheumatoid arthritis, which she recalls was a huge relief.

Becoming increasingly interested in resolving pain rather than just managing it, Georgie trained in Reflexology and Adapted Reflextherapy in spinal pain, along with a specific type of Bowen Therapy called Neurostructural Integration Technique, and set up her own private clinic. Through all of these techniques, she became aware of how important it was to treat the patient holistically rather than as a set of symptoms or a body part.

Viewing and treating a patient holistically was encouraged when I was a student though at times it feels like 'holistic' is almost a dirty word within the medical world. I think this is short-sighted and we are missing a trick when we don't use it to our advantage. A holistic approach can tell us so much and we are much more likely to help the patient get a good outcome. In addition to this, taking the holistic view helps you connect with patients (and other healthcare professionals) more than if you just see them as a 'knee' or 'the nurse you work with who happens to be in a bad mood', so it is a win-win really!

In addition to noticing anomalies with patients' symptoms that didn't fit the normal pain pattern and becoming frustrated with the traditional medical model approach, Georgie herself developed severe sciatica. She had no injury or predisposing factors to attribute it to. It soon became clear to her that it was related to the stress she was feeling due to setting up her own business and not having a regular salary.

At this time she came across the work of Dr John Sarno. He is a rehabilitation specialist in New York who has been doing pioneering work since the 1970s, theorising that repressed emotions can trigger the unconscious part of the nervous system to create pain, which becomes a distraction from the underlying cause. He suggests that if the cause is dealt with properly then the pain can be resolved. His theories have polarised opinion.

By reading Dr Sarno's books and following his advice, Georgie resolved all her symptoms over the next few months as she came to understand how many of them were stress induced in some way. She went from having some form of treatment every two or three months for various recurring symptoms to having none at all and feeling fitter than ever. At the end of 2007, Georgie decided to fly to the US to spend some time with Dr Sarno to find out more. This helped her answer questions about the confusion she had experienced with the presentation of her patients' symptoms and enabled her to set up her own patient programme in the UK. As a specialist in this field, Georgie trains other practitioners in an approach which has education and self-empowerment at its core.

So can stress really cause so many problems? Let's remind ourselves of the effects of stress on the body - see illustration on the following page.

Stress

Stress is crafty; it sneaks up on you when you are looking in the opposite direction or when you are busy.

We are experiencing a stress epidemic in the developed world. We are bombarded by so much information that our senses have to process, we rarely have a chance to do nothing and just be. We forget that:

*'We are human **beings** not human **doings**.'*

Effects of stress on the body

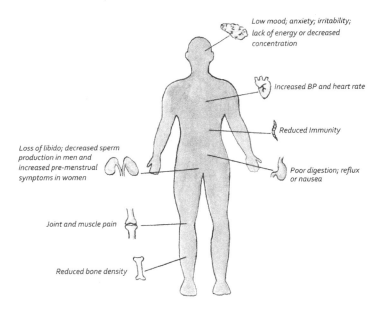

We are all so used to the fast pace of our lives these days that we often don't recognise how stressed we feel. As healthcare professionals I think that we can be especially guilty of this because we constantly focus on others and fail to tune in to ourselves. Stress becomes normal as we 'cope' with what's happening in our lives and often suppress our own issues.

During your first years working in the health professions it is common to experience high levels of stress and anxiety. We have all been there. As a student you have what seem like never-ending exams and clinical placements. You feel like you are being tested in new environments all the time. When you finish university you rejoice that you are now qualified – then the pressure goes up a notch and you are subjected to new stresses and pressures (often many that are self-imposed!). You care; you want to do a good job. You berate yourself for being less than perfect or remember the one thing that didn't go well. The hours and paperwork sap your energy and stop you doing what you came into the profession to do.

Georgie also knows how this feels and remarks:

'I never realized how much stress I was actually causing myself. Self-talk [negative] was having a huge impact on me, yet I had no idea. It's often said that 10% of our perceived stress is what is actually happening and the other 90% is how we respond to it and I began to realise that most of my health issues were a result of that. Realising who I am, and why I am who I am as a result of my past experiences, also helped me then work on this.'

Georgie helped me realise that negative emotions directed at yourself are as harmful as feeling angry with someone else. I think that, as healthcare professionals, this is quite common amongst us. We tend to be perfectionists with high expectations of ourselves and we like to be in control. These personality traits can push us to be high achievers, but they can also be detrimental. Personality plays a huge part in how we react to what's happening around us and we tend to ignore these self-induced pressures which can lead to significant stress.

To help you understand how stress affects your body, we need to look a little deeper at what happens at a physiological level.

The wonderful autonomic nervous system

The Autonomic Nervous System (ANS) is part of the nervous system we learn about at university but we can have a tendency to neglect it when we try to understand and diagnose symptoms.

The ANS beavers away automatically without requiring conscious effort. Made up of two branches (the *Parasympathetic* and the *Sympathetic*) the ANS strives to maintain homeostasis in the body. Most organs are supplied by both the sympathetic and parasympathetic branches (except for the skin which is only supplied by the sympathetic side).

Autonomic Nervous System

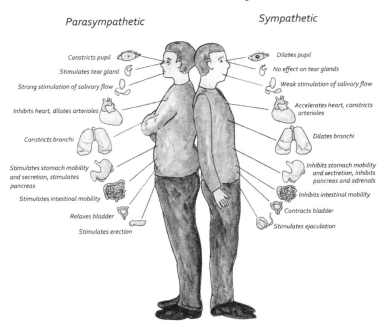

Effects on the body by the two sections of the autonomic nervous system

When stress causes stimulation of the sympathetic side, it results in increased secretion of multiple neurotransmitters (including *epinephrine* and *norepinephrine*). Even neural circuitry is reallocated. Cortisol is secreted from the adrenal gland and causes suppression of the immune system. Noradrenaline (Nor Ad) increases respiratory rate, increases heart rate, increases muscle contraction and affects the liver. Nor Ad also affects the hypothalamus, which in turn affects the pituitary, then the adrenal cortex. This can all lead to a whole host of signs and symptoms:

Signs of Sympathetic nervous system (SNS) over-activation:
- Sweating hands
- Increased neural tension or neural tension tests produce sweating
- Emotional: anxiety; depression; moody; irritability; feeling overwhelmed or panic attacks
- Cognitive: poor memory; worrying; inability to concentrate or make decisions
- Physical: pain; bowel problems
- Behavioural: eating and sleeping more or less; using alcohol, cigarettes or drugs to relax; withdrawal socially

Symptoms of SNS over-activation:
- Sweating
- Chronic pain
- Nausea
- Loss of memory
- Decreased ability to sequence thoughts
- Feels as if insects crawling over legs, face

- Water running down legs
- Patient may feel they are going loopy
- Mental and physical dysfunction
- Tiredness
- Emotional; tearful

Connective tissue is also innervated by the SNS, with the exception of cartilage; therefore, whatever is happening in the SNS will affect the connective tissue. This also backs up the mind-body connection and the fact that stress can indeed affect physical structures.

We learn about this magic system academically and never really in relation to stress. As healthcare professionals we are aware of stress but we ignore it and forget simple physiology as evidence that the mind and body are interconnected. Patients can get caught in an adrenaline-run SNS, keeping them in the fight/flight response. They become unable to get out of it and have no idea how they could. As healthcare professionals, we should know better but we also get stuck in this loop.

Chronic stress

If stress is extreme or long lasting, even at a low level, the normal coping mechanisms of the body fail. Often the body's immune system and ability to resist disease can be compromised severely. I had chronic low-level stress and that is why I kept getting ill, though it took me a long time to realise the connection. My body kept telling me that there was something wrong, that something needed to change, but I kept ignoring it.

I had a few episodes of really bad nausea when I was a

junior physio. It would come on for no reason and it really put me off food (anyone who knows me will recognise that this is pretty serious as I love food and love to cook!). I also had episodes of a heavy mental fog during which time I just didn't feel myself or felt I wasn't quite present. I would also have this frustrating post-viral type fatigue when I had had a cold which would drag on for a few weeks. As a student I also recall having a week (in hindsight it was just before a stressful exam) of dreadful night sweats and a couple of emotional episodes when I was just crying all the time for no reason.

A few years ago when I was going through a relationship break-up I developed random pain in my left thumb. As a physio I thought that I should be able to diagnose myself. It presented as a painful clicking in my left MCP joint in the thumb – horrible, though it went immediately. The pain lasted for a few weeks until I realised that there was an emotional reason and after addressing the cause with some stream of consciousness writing (see Chapter 8) it disappeared.

I also developed embarrassing facial blushing when I started a new job a few years ago. I had never had this before and it was not related to situations where I would normally have been embarrassed. I put it down to working in a new environment that was maybe challenging me on a level different from before. On reflection, it was also during the period when I was very stressed in my relationship and not facing up to things. It was resolved completely when I dealt with the underlying issue and I have not suffered since.

I am not a doctor, I am a physio but I have learned over the years to tune in to my body. I believe that my symptoms were definitely related to over activation of the SNS. Obviously I would advise anyone with physical symptoms to get checked out medically to rule out any other condition.

You need not only to become more self-aware but to allow yourself to have compassion towards your symptoms. What are they trying to tell you? Are they telling you that you are stressed, or struggling with an emotional issue? Can you identify any symptoms that you have or have had in the past? What are your stressors? How can you avoid or limit them, or how can you look at them differently? Sometimes just making these links can help you resolve the symptoms or prevent a recurrence.

We often accept stress and ignore symptoms but this can be dangerous; it doesn't just cause the stimulation of the SNS but, more crucially, involves the abatement of the parasympathetic nervous system (PNS). What can we do to reverse this and enhance the PNS side?

The soothing nature of compassion

If you are constantly in fight or flight mode (in an over activated SNS state) then it is impossible for you to be in a truly compassionate state, where attributes such as calmness, peace and forgiveness are important.

The experience of compassion evokes responses within the human body that awaken the PNS, soothing the effects of the stress response and over-stimulation of the SNS. Caring relationships cause a decrease in SNS activity by the effects of *oxytocin* and *vasopressin*.

Released from the hypothalamus, oxytocin decreases the hypothalamic-pituitary-adrenal axis (a complex set of interactions between the hypothalamus, the pituitary and the adrenal glands, this is a major part of the neuroendocrine system that controls stress and regulates many body processes) and increases PNS activity.

The actions of the magic hormone oxytocin (which you can now buy as an oral spray supplement!) have been shown to decrease blood pressure and reduce stress. Oxytocin is known as the trust or love chemical as it induces feelings of happiness, contentedness and closeness. It is also seen to decrease pain and even act as an anti-depressant.

Ways to increase oxytocin:
- Hugging
- Touch
- Watch a tear-jerker film
- Sing or dance (with others)
- Do something scary or thrilling with someone
- Anything that increases connections – even Facebook (though better in person)

Because of the connection between the mind and the body, if you treat the nervous system, you will in turn treat and strengthen the immune system. Begin to recognise how your own personality and stressors may affect you.

Georgie's top tips

1. Recognise how you speak to yourself. Do you find yourself blaming, being self-critical and over-analytical? If so, learn ways to address this, such as being mindful; reframing what has happened; developing a feeling of gratitude or distracting yourself with something fun, mentally stimulating or that involves social connections.
2. Write a journal to offload how you feel now or how

you felt during a traumatic/emotional time in the past. Allow yourself to be the victim while you do this but then look at things from another perspective in order to understand, accept and let them go. This isn't always easy and as Georgie says, 'People will only change when the pain of changing is less than the pain of not changing'.
3. Self-care: love yourself first. You have to put yourself first, so do something for yourself each week.
4. It's alright to show vulnerability.
5. Find time to be still each day, maybe sitting quietly with no distractions, going for a walk or meditating. Even if you can't take thirty minutes to meditate or sit quietly, spend two minutes hiding in the toilet and ground yourself.

Dealing with trauma and grief

PROFESSOR GORDON TURNBULL is a world leader in the field of trauma; he has motivated a change in the field of mental health, particularly in respect to Post Traumatic Stress Disorder (PTSD) in the armed forces. I met Gordon some seven years ago thanks to him using a room within the physiotherapy department I worked in. He had a very open referral process between the physiotherapy department and his speciality as a psychiatrist which meant that we could ask him for advice about patients or refer them to him for further help.

Gordon has led a fascinating life following his passion which began in medical school at Edinburgh University before joining the Royal Air Force (RAF). Choosing to pursue a path in psychiatry after his illusions about becoming a surgeon were shattered by a rather bullish superior, he was drawn into the field of psychological trauma. His experience has been wide reaching: he was involved directly after the Lockerbie air disaster; he was as psychiatric advisor during the Gulf War of 1991, and he conducted the first-ever debriefings of British prisoners of war and British hostages released from Lebanon. He is also dedicated to trauma services for police officers, emergency service personnel, military veterans and civilians. He is now consultant psychiatrist in trauma at Capio Nightingale Hospitals in London, advisor in psychiatry to the Civil Aviation Authority and professor at the University of Chester. He has pushed the boundaries in medicine and challenged a lot of previously ingrained thoughts, working tirelessly in getting PTSD recognised as a condition.

What has it got to do with my patients?

You may be wondering what trauma has to do with treating a patient with a broken leg or nursing an elderly man on a hospital ward. It has everything to do with it.

As healthcare professionals, we see many patients who have suffered some form of trauma though the signs may be very subtle; they may be presenting with something quite different. Our job is to be a detective at times and not always take symptoms at face value.

We forget that we need to help patients deal with every aspect of their recovery. If we can't offer direct help then we can always offer a compassionate ear and a kind touch that will help release oxytocin in them and us.

When Gordon released his book *Trauma: From Lockerbie to 7/7 – How Trauma Affects Our Minds and How We Fight Back*, I knew that I had to read it because I knew him and was fascinated with this topic. I wasn't disappointed; his gentle manner comes across in his writing which highlights how trauma can affect us all. It caused me to reflect on patients I have seen whom I feel I could have helped more, often because I lacked awareness of how much the mind can influence the body or vice versa.

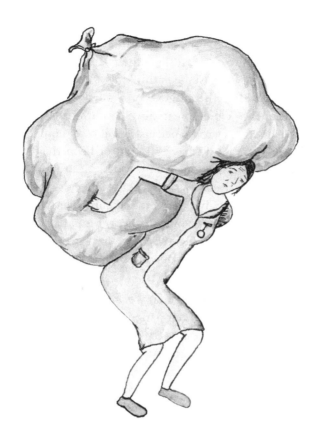

Relevance to you as an individual

Watching or imagining other people experiencing pain activates your central nervous systems pain matrix. The brain is unable to tell if something is real or not; consequently you can suffer from hearing about an event even though you haven't experienced it.

Some healthcare professionals seem to believe that you just need to toughen up and become hardened to the emotional side of patient contact as a way of avoiding being affected by other people's trauma. Indeed, sometimes distance is needed; it would not be great to have a surgeon falling apart in the operating theatre because he is thinking about how sore the patient will be after the surgery, or a nurse unable to deal with a patient in a life-threatening condition needing her help in the emergency room because she is over-empathising. However, as patients we have all seen or been treated by a healthcare professional who is a bit too blunt or emotionally removed from the situation. You feel that they don't care and that can be very damaging to the therapeutic relationship. As a healthcare professional you can't expect a patient to open up to you if you are distant; they may even play down their symptoms. So we need to be open to patients but at the same time we need to protect ourselves.

We also need to be aware that we are affected by our own traumas as well as those of our patient's. We are often so busy being caring, putting on our professional identity along with our uniforms, that we forget that we don't always have to be the superhero. Trauma inevitably affects us too and we need to learn to ask for help in these situations.

'One of the biggest obstacles in nursing [and other healthcare professions] is not allowing ourselves to grieve and supporting one another as well as recognizing our dysfunctional methods of dealing with the feelings we keep burying.'

(Ewing & Carter, 2005)

As a nineteen-year-old student, just prior to my oncology placement, both my grandmother and grandfather died within a few months of each other; my grandfather had been diagnosed with lung cancer. I hardly told anyone about this at the time; I thought I should also be able to cope with what was going on in my personal life. In hindsight, believing that I should put my personal emotions to one side when I was the *professional* on placement only made things worse. At the time I didn't make the connection between my sense of loss when a patient died and my grief for my grandparents. I was not taught at university how things in your own life will affect your ability to cope at work. I have since learned the importance of dealing with my own trauma rather than ignoring it. Although it sometimes feels like the latter is easier, it is not healthy in the long run.

My career path took me in a similar direction to Gordon's after I took a locum physiotherapy post with the military. I could not have worked in this area a few years ago as I don't think that I could have coped with the patients and their problems, or not without getting ill again myself. Working in this area has been fascinating and very rewarding but not without its challenges. I have become acutely aware of how important it is to tune into myself when I am dealing with trauma patients whose minds are influencing their physical symptoms.

So what actually happens in trauma and how is it different to stress?

What actually happens in trauma?

There are many causes that can lead to trauma:
- Car accident
- Abuse
- Mugging, burglary or act of violence
- Injury or severe illness
- Bereavement
- Natural disaster

I am not going to attempt to unravel the intricacies of what happens in trauma or how to treat trauma (I am not a psychiatrist!). Gordon does so eloquently in his book, defining it as a survival tool that is a:

'Normal reaction, in normal people to an abnormal event.'

Trauma is similar to the over-activation of the SNS that happens when the body is subjected to stress, though it appears to go a few levels further with the centre responsible for speech (Broca's area) beginning to shut down and also the area responsible for experiencing what happens in the present moment (medial prefrontal cortex) shutting down.

This often results in hyperarousal which can present as:
- Depression of mood
- Increased anxiety; hyperarousal or panic attacks
- Deterioration of memory and concentration
- Anger or emotional outbursts
- Irritability
- Lethargy/fatigue

How can we help deal with trauma and resolve it?

We have to choose our own path in life as to whether we deal with traumas, and when we are ready to deal with them. There is no single recipe for dealing with them, just like there is no one recipe for dealing with a patient with a certain set of symptoms. Everyone is different and everyone needs something different in terms of help.

Whether we offer our patients tools, if they are ready

for them, or whether we work on ourselves, acknowledging there is a problem is a start.

Verbalising trauma

Speaking about a traumatic event can have strong physiological effects that impact on both mental and physical health. I know from my experience as a student physiotherapist that if I had been encouraged to talk about my personal grief and also that of experiencing the death of patients, I may have been able to process it, understand it and deal with it better. Historically this has been an alien concept in most of the healthcare profession; we learn to cope and believe that we should be able to cope.

I have a friend who is a psychologist who has regular counselling and debrief sessions as part of her role (something that all psychologists and counsellors seem to do). Why do most other healthcare professionals not think that this is necessary and instead expect to cope by ourselves?

Thankfully this attitude is slowly beginning to shift. I came across the concept of 'Schwartz Rounds' a few years ago which were being piloted at the Royal Free Hospital in London. These meetings are a practical way of discussing the emotional impact of the work we do as healthcare professionals. They can provide an open forum for discussion of the decision-making process and act as an effective means of stress reduction by allowing staff to talk about difficult situations. The concept of these meetings originated in the US.

The session that I witnessed was a great example of multiple healthcare disciplines coming together to discuss and share their experiences of trauma. It was led by the team whose job it is to answer all the cardiac arrest calls in the hospital. They had developed effective ways to support and debrief each other which they realised were imperative in their roles. They had noticed how this help and support was not available to other healthcare professionals and how traumatic these events were for them. It was refreshing to hear them talk about how dealing with the effects of trauma was important. This kind of awareness and sharing how our experiences with patients can deeply affect us as healthcare professionals needs to be addressed. I am pleased to see that there are now around 100 health and care organisations in the UK which are contracted to run Schwartz Rounds (see the resource section for further details).

I learned the value of counselling a few years ago when I was going through a particularly stressful time in my personal life. I learned that you have to be prepared to be vulnerable in order to address issues, though in order to do this you must be able to connect with the healthcare professional. After a couple of sessions with a counsellor who had been recommended to me, I started making feeble excuses as to why I couldn't make the next appointment we had scheduled. I knew that I didn't have the right connection with her and I was never going to open up because of this. Finding another counsellor who was the right fit made all the difference. I learned so much from this experience and I am not ashamed to talk about it. I learned that it was OK to ask for and ultimately accept help, despite being a healthcare practitioner myself.

Counselling is often thought of as the main approach in treating trauma, grief or in dealing with stress. However, techniques that focus more on the body can be a good alternative as the root of our experiences is often stored deeply in the body.

Body approaches

The body-oriented or 'somatic' approach focuses on using the bodily symptoms that may be observed in trauma and teaching various body techniques instead of the use of counselling. It has been argued that due to the overload placed on the nervous system during trauma, it needs to be addressed through the body before the emotions can be fully processed.

'The somatic approach can radically alter the body's physiology. It can rewire your brain and change the fear system in your brain. It can regulate the balance between the SNS and the PNS and activate the cranial nerves so your body doesn't respond to everything as if it is getting hurt.'

Van der Kolk

Body techniques:
- Somatic experiencing
- Trauma Releasing Exercises (TRE)
- Yoga
- Sensory motor therapy
- Eye Movement and Desensitisation Reprocessing (EMDR)
- Hakomi method
- Cardiac Coherence Technique – a type of breathing technique

(See Chapter 8 for further details of these techniques)

An advantage that these body techniques can have over talking or counselling is that emotional wounds can be too painful to discuss. Also, the emotional effects of the trauma may not be on a conscious level and so you (or your patient) may have trouble articulating them.

Increasingly practitioners are using talking-type therapies in conjunction with body techniques. Like any treatment technique, there cannot be a prescriptive formula that we can follow. I benefited from having counselling but throughout that time I was also exercising and doing yoga, so I was actually combining the two techniques.

Being prepared to share your vulnerability with friends, colleagues and even patients can have immeasurable benefits. Sometimes as healthcare professionals we need to put up our hands and not to be afraid to say that we are not coping. Far from being a sign of weakness, I feel that this takes great courage and can lead to personal development and improve your health. Sharing yourself with patients or colleagues can allow you to gain more of a connection. Don't be scared that people will judge you.

Gordon's top tips

1. A question from a consultant physician when I had little experience was: *'If you had only thirty minutes with a patient, would you split your time 50/50 or would you take longer to examine or longer to take history?'* The answer he gave was to take twenty-five minutes for the history and then five to examine. This is something I always remembered and taught me the importance of listening to the story behind the symptoms.
2. Some people can be quite awkward. Seeing them objectively, without getting entangled with them, is the best way forward.

3. To be empathetic doesn't always involve talking; become a good listener. Sometimes patients just need someone to listen.
4. Maintain compassion by not becoming too involved and by regarding the patient's problem as being a solution that you need to find together. Recognise the difference between yourself and the other person, then you can make objective decisions about what they need.
5. Self-care is important and helps to replenish your energy. For Gordon this includes: going to the pub on a Friday; using a Microcurrent machine (see references) to rebalance himself; spending time engaging with the outside world and watching comedies or murder mysteries.

It's all about feel!

DOUG NEWBURG IS an inspiring, though slightly unconventional (by his own reckoning), sport psychologist whom I came across when I was undertaking my MSc in Sport Psychology. I spent the first semester telling my supervisor that I definitely wasn't going to do the research part of the MSc as I had bad memories of research from my undergraduate days. I found the research process dry, stressful and unrelated to the clinical practice that I enjoyed so much. I also hated statistics and still didn't understand them when I was finished! I understood the importance of research but I couldn't fully engage with it.

Then I came across Doug's work and the research that had been done using his work; immediately it made sense and I was hooked. The concept of resonance 'resonated' with me when I first heard about it. I read about how Doug had worked with hundreds of sports people and interviewed more than 600 top-level performers in music, business and sport in order to answer questions about whether these high-performing people have something in common. His answer was *feel*.

After gaining valuable personal experience playing basketball, and empathy for what it feels like to be on the bench, Doug decided to go back to university to get his PhD in Sport Psychology. He found that athletes, and others, who had been through similar experiences to himself were better at answering his questions than those in the academic world. Since then he has spent years learning about performance and seeking out people who have inspired him. He came to understand that these people did not distinguish between how they lived and how they performed – one was feeding the other.

How do you want to feel each day?

People forget why they went into the healthcare professions. Every person Doug interviewed told him that remembering *why* you are doing your work is important. It creates energy when your physical energy is spent. All of Doug's findings support what Salmaan and others also encourage: to remember why you do what you do. Doug has also spent time with medical students encouraging them to recall why they went into medicine in the first place.

'Happiness is feeling the way you like to feel.'

Remembering the reason you went into the healthcare professions is important; getting in touch with how it makes you feel … and then working out how you get to feel this every day is the next challenge. What can you influence and have an effect on? You can certainly take responsibility for how you *want* to feel each day and start to notice whether you are feeling anywhere close to this. Beginning to understand these things, not settling for the fact that you are busy and thus have not done what makes you feel good is the first step.

Doug is a great teacher and practices what he preaches,

advising that you need to allow time for the things you enjoy, both inside and outside work. He suggests that you should find people who you want to learn from, observe, ask questions of, as well as learning to listen to your own life. Building his life around feel, he loves being on his bike and has even learned to love how riding uphill makes him feel!

I have learned that paying attention to feel was one of the missing links for me. Feeling energised, open and relaxed allows me to be more giving. Setting my intentions for the day as I drive to work opens my frame of reference and allows me to take charge of how I want to feel. Exercising at lunchtimes makes a huge difference to how I feel for the rest of the day. Knowing that I have spent some time on myself makes me more able to give to others. It also gives me the headspace to switch from work mode for a while, not to mention releasing all those lovely endorphins! At the end of each day, I also spend a few moments in bed thinking about what I am grateful for.

How you feel matters greatly, as it forces you to look at and respond to obstacles inside of you rather than only dealing with external problems. You need to reconnect with yourself in dealings with patients and be self-aware in this whole process ... it is not just about the patient. I have learned through doing my research and working with patients to trust what feels right.

To begin to understand how you would like to feel, you need to become aware of yourself. As you start to do this, don't expect that you will immediately know how you want to feel. It is not necessarily a cognitive process.

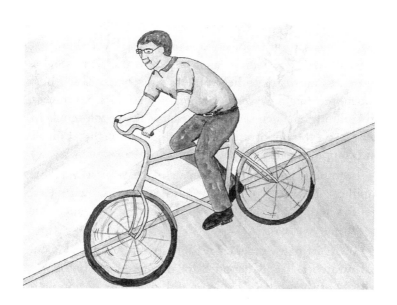

Becoming aware of yourself

Awareness of yourself is the first step towards helping yourself. How you deal with other people, the things they tell you and the things you hear can affect you enormously. It is so easy to get caught up by external factors rather than connecting with ourselves. I know only too well that we often lack awareness of our physical and emotional needs as healthcare professionals. It can feel selfish or self-indulgent to think about ourselves before the patient or client who is in front of us, asking for help.

Who is going to help the patient if we are ill or feeling so exhausted that we have to present an armoured wall to protect ourselves? If we are not self-aware, it can lead to a self-destructive pattern of overwork. All of this makes it so easy to lose touch with why we are doing the job we used to love, experience more stress and less empathy, and have a greater likelihood of developing empathy fatigue.

Self-awareness involves a combination of knowing yourself and developing a *split awareness*. This double awareness allows us to help others with compassion whilst also monitoring how we are feeling. Increased self-awareness, and offering as much care for yourself as the people you help, allows you the opportunity to remain emotionally available and compassionate even in the most stressful situations.

Becoming more self-aware can make your work more fulfilling. It can also allow you to re-connect with your passion and gift for helping others, whilst at the same time nurturing yourself.

There are many practical ways that you can increase your self-awareness (see Chapter 8 for more details). Before we talk about them, spend some time thinking about how self-aware you are. Do you notice anything about yourself when you are with patients/clients? Is it positive or negative? Or are you so focused on the other person you have no idea how you feel until the end of a session/end of the day?

How you feel affects whether you just survive the day or whether you begin to flourish.

Reflection

Central to Doug's concept of resonance and feel is the process of reflection. Reflection is very powerful and can lead to greater self-awareness. It relies on openness, honesty and trust.

As a physiotherapy student, I was encouraged to do reflective writing and I quite enjoyed it (maybe I was a bit of a nerd!). As a practising healthcare professional, it is something that is encouraged within our Continuing

Professional Development (CPD) though at times it can feel like something that needs to be done rather than something that you really want to do.

I didn't fully appreciate the value of reflection until I undertook my MSc. It made me realise that as a student it can help you to ground you. It also allows you to deal with feelings associated with the experiences you have. Essentially it helps you understand other people and, most importantly, yourself. It helps you when otherwise you wouldn't be able to see the wood for the trees, when you are overwhelmed emotionally and when you simply don't understand what happened or why you reacted in a certain way. Reflecting on what you have done well, what aspects of work you enjoy and when you are happiest are all important. It is easy to focus on your weaknesses or on what didn't go well rather than on your strengths.

Reflection can be a very beneficial process at a personal level and facilitate self-development; at the same time it can make you feel vulnerable as it often means stepping outside your comfort zone. I have learned to tune in to my feelings more. When I am feeling anxious or stressed, I ask myself why and try to unravel the feeling so that I can see what I can do about it.

Reflective writing has really helped me not only develop as a professional but also, and more importantly, personally. Writing this book has caused me to reflect on the signs and symptoms that I have had over the years and previously dismissed or ignored.

Once you know how you want to feel and how you can get this feeling during the day, you need to think about how you connect with others.

Making connections

As humans we are all searching for connections and we all want to connect with others in some way; it makes us feel understood and valued. Maybe as healthcare professionals we need this because of our personality types. Doug agrees that we often confuse *attachment* with *connection*. With compassion we are looking for connection ... instead we sometimes create attachments. The difference between connection and attachment:

'Attachment is like you are on the phone with somebody and they hang up their end but you never hang up your end of the phone because you are waiting for them to pick the phone back up, they don't and then you think there is something wrong with you when they don't. Connection is when you have the conversation and you say everything that needs to be said, two-way and equal.'

This attachment can cause some negative feelings that we suffer as healthcare professionals. We start taking on others' problems. You can feel like you have failed as a professional as you take on too much and begin to experience what the patient feels.

Another setback in making genuine connections at times can in fact be our training. We are encouraged to become the 'expert', which can be great for our sense of professional identity and give us confidence. However, it can have a detrimental effect on the connections we try to make with not only our patients but other healthcare professionals.

Our training can separate us from those who we really need to connect with, suggesting that we are the professional and they are the patient and therefore different. We also separate ourselves from other healthcare professionals by distinguishing ourselves as different by the uniforms we wear and our different agendas. We forget that we are the same and that we are all working towards the same goal, to help the patient.

We all agree that the patient's story is important and I understand the reason for an emphasis on patient-centred care but I wonder whether there should be a shift towards team-centred care, with the patient being an equal member of the team. Within this team everyone needs to respect each other but also to respect themselves as an integral part of the team; this is often much harder. How the patient feels is important but how you feel is more important. In order to be able to take care of your patient you need to respect, look after and understand how you feel.

'Our deepest fear is not that we are inadequate. Our deepest fear is that we are powerful beyond measure. It is our light, not our darkness, that most frightens us. We ask ourselves, who am I to be brilliant, gorgeous, talented and fabulous? Actually, who are you not to be? Your playing small doesn't serve the world. There's nothing enlightened about shrinking so that other people won't feel insecure around you. We were born to make manifest the glory that is within us. It is not just in some of us; it's in everyone. And as we let our own light shine, we unconsciously give other people permission to do the same. As we are liberated from our own fear, our presence automatically liberates others.'

Nelson Mandela

Doug's top tips

1. Take responsibility for how you feel. Do you like being yourself? Have you built the things that you can count on (things that make you feel better if you are feeling bad)? People don't value 'feel' and don't take responsibility for it. Caregivers think that taking care of other people is going to make them feel the way they like to feel but then they realise that it doesn't.
2. Living what makes you happy rather than chasing what you want.
3. Discussion groups – we need to be vulnerable and trust, to allow ourselves to be human. Share the positive stuff, not just the negative, with each other.
4. Reflective writing.
5. Don't keep doing the same thing over and over and expecting a different result.

Being Mindful

RICK HANSON IS a leader in the mindfulness field and someone whom I have admired and followed from afar. He is an influential teacher whose kindness and passion shines through in his approach to wellness and his mindful approach to compassion.

As a neuropsychologist, Rick has written and taught about personal well-being, psychological growth and contemplative practice. After doing a variety of jobs (even for a mathematician, working out the probability of a nuclear power plant melting down!) he did a near-masters in Developmental Psychology. He shifted towards clinical training midway through his thesis when he realised he wanted to be a therapist more than a professor. This was followed by a PhD in Clinical Psychology. Working with individual clients, he has also had considerable involvement with schools, consulting as a psychologist for several independent schools. Over the years he became increasingly interested in the connection between modern brain science and ancient contemplative practices and founded the Wellspring Institute for Neuroscience and Contemplative Wisdom. Rick is also a Senior Fellow of the Greater Good Science Centre at UC Berkeley and the author of a number of articles. He has written many practical books which guide us how to change our brain to help relieve stress, reduce worry and live better.

Being mindful about compassion

Although compassion comes naturally to most of us who go into the healthcare professions, it often requires some intention to be maintained. Rick has over time cultivated recognition in himself of the profound value of compassion, the benefits for himself and the benefits for others. This has been a process which he feels he has actively cultivated: taking in moments of compassion, tending to compassion and as a result become more compassionate.

'The more caring and empathic you are by nature and the more caring and empathic you become by training, the more important it is to develop boundaries. They too can be cultivated over time.'

A lot is talked about the fine balance between compassion and equanimity, where on the one hand we are open to the suffering of others and on the other hand we do not suffer as a result. Logically this makes total sense but achieving it can be hard.

I know this first hand. I used to pick up on what my patients were feeling; they would feel much better but I would be exhausted and drained! I learned over time that this was not healthy for me, or sustainable, and I got to the point where I felt that I couldn't remain empathetic. At times I felt like there was no barrier and I didn't know how to stop absorbing other people's emotions. I was inviting it in by asking them about themselves and was extremely sensitive to their emotions. Rick highlights the importance of realising that their suffering is not your suffering; a patient's suffering should not make you suffer.

Have you ever worked with people who you feel are a negative influence on you or who sap your energy? Do you have any patients, colleagues or friends who leave you feeling exhausted after you have spoken with them?

I have learned the hard way that it is important to protect yourself from these influences as they can have a negative effect on your health especially if you are a compassionate/empathic person. It doesn't mean that you have to become stand-offish; you just need the ability to recognise these people and how to deal with them.

Some people can drain the life blood out of you. They are a bit like the *dementors* in Harry Potter – getting too near them can suck the positive, happy feeling out of you. It is a bit like a mist that descends over things and if you are sensitive to it, you may feel depressed or exhausted after you have encountered these people … when they usually feel better!

Instead of judging them, recognise that there may be reasons why they are like this. Also recognise that spending all your energy, either listening, observing or reacting to what they say may be counterproductive. Some people like to get a reaction from others; sometimes they have no idea that how they act or what they say has an effect on others.

Part of self-compassion is being aware that you may be more sensitive to these people. You may not feel anything at the time but hours later you feel stressed, low or exhausted. Self-compassion in this context is about being kind to yourself and understanding what you need in these situations. You may need to let the things that are being said wash over you or you may need to remove yourself politely from the situation.

We all have different tolerance levels and different levels of sensitivity. Sometimes, particularly if we are feeling tired, low or ill, our tolerance levels for these people are reduced – recognise this.

You cannot influence what others say and do, you can only control how you react to them. Take time to protect yourself and recognise times when you are vulnerable.

Being in any of the health/caring professions can be painful and tiring, but it also must be rewarding and sustaining for us to survive!

'It takes dedication, hard disciplined work, and intensive training before a dancer can move with unearthly grace and perform feats that are impossible for an untrained body. In the same way, people have found that when they practice compassion assiduously, all day and every day, they achieve new capacities of mind and heart.'

Karen Armstrong

To Rick, it all comes down to a sense of presence. Being mindful is about an awareness of your present state. Being able to generate a sense of awareness within your own body naturally tends to differentiate you from other people. It allows you to really care for your patient but not be invaded or depleted by them. If we are disturbed or frustrated, it is hard to access compassion for ourselves and for others.

Mindfulness is about being in the moment, whether it is taking a moment to look out of the window at the world outside, taking time to enjoy lunch or really being present with a patient. Research in healthcare professionals shows that mindfulness and sustained present moment awareness can help to reduce burnout.

Being aware applies not only to being aware of how you like to feel but also how you *don't* like to feel. Take time to tune into how you feel and how everyday things can push you away from how you want to feel. Take moments to reflect throughout the day on how you can soothe your emotions, or take time to enjoy the little things. These moments can do wonders for your health!

'I am very good at taking in the good. I really try to look for those little moments each day where I accomplish something or I make contact with someone.'

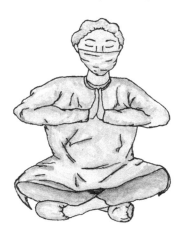

Meditation and neuroplasticity

Meditating can help you centre, be present and consider the bigger picture. Even a few minutes a day can have profound effects on your physiology as well as increasing self-awareness and awareness of others. Meditation activates the 'compassion' area of the brain (anterior insular cortex). Neuroscientific research from the Met Sinai Medical Centre in New York has discovered that when the brain is scanned during meditation, the empathy area lights up significantly. Meditation also increases self-awareness and awareness of others.

Rick meditates every day, committing to a minute or more (usually a lot more!). Meditation for him is one form of personal renewal – though he has others as well; he joked that he may use a trip to the bathroom to read a page from a novel as a chance for him to reset.

'Reading was a refuge for me in my family when I was growing up and so it takes me back to my childhood.'

I have done some meditation, though I admit that I find guided meditation much easier than trying to sit and empty my mind. Through yoga I have tried different types of meditation that may be easier if you are a new student. Alternate nostril breathing and square breathing are two techniques I have outlined in the practical skills section (Chapter 8) for you to try.

Your unconscious mind is very open to suggestion when you are in a relaxed state so listening to a guided imagery meditation is a great way to imbed some positive affirmations.

I have been lucky enough to use some of the skills I learned on my MSc course and teach relaxation sessions to patients. I have seen how much physical and mental benefit yoga and relaxation can have on severely injured and disabled patients. I often wonder why we are open enough to do this with patients and not with ourselves or each other during a staff session.

Neuroplasticity occurs when there is prolonged activity in one part of the brain. Meditation and mindfulness are ways that we can influence our brains and change how we think. I used to roll my eyes at university when the term 'neuroplasticity' was mentioned; it is ironic that I now think it is amazing!

As healthcare professionals, we understand neuroplasticity in relation to patients and in particular within neurology, such as in those who have had a stroke. We rarely associate neuroplasticity with ourselves. We have so much more control over what we think than we realise.

Changing what you can change

As healthcare professionals we have all wondered why our work can't be less demanding, less stressful and less depleting. It would be great if there was less pressure on meeting targets and fewer restrictions on how we work. It would be great to feel that we could offer every patient what we wanted to offer. I am an optimist but I also understand that this is not the world we live in within the healthcare environment.

Rick suggests that if you are going to pour out a lot, you have GOT to fill up your own cup! You have got to take care of yourself and you have to take time, even if it is just a few minutes in the bathroom to 'reset' or having realistic expectations of what you can actually do today.

'Really look for those moments (10, 30 or 60 secs at a time) where you can reset yourself, come back to centre. Splash some water on your face; eat something sweet; touch someone that you care about; make a joke; lift your eyes up to the horizon line (which helps us see the big picture neurologically); exhale slowly and feel the relaxing of your breath; think of something you feel grateful for or something that is beautiful.'

The state and private health systems all have flaws that frustrate us. Unfortunately the system does not care about us as individual workers or how we feel. The values of this system are often disconnected with what you value as a healthcare professional. I think that the system has partly been why I have moved around in my work and why at times I used to come home feeling incredibly frustrated.

As Rick points out, doctors are often closer to the top in terms of the power. I have watched them on many occasions where they can command what they want, sometimes without much care for the patient let alone other healthcare professionals. On the other hand, nurses and other health professionals can feel a strong sense of helplessness, futility and powerlessness.

It is a vicious circle as this helplessness can cause you to feel low in mood, more frustrated and exhausted. The physical exhaustion then makes you feel less motivated to stay in the profession. (I know that this varies depending on the person, and can affect doctors as well as other healthcare professionals.)

To survive and eventually flourish in the system, you must take care of yourself so that you don't burn out or wear down your ability to care. You can take little opportunities to take back your power. Notice ways in which you are having a beneficial impact on someone. Sometimes this is hard and feels quite alien. I had to change the way I was conditioned and learn that taking care of my own needs was ABSOLUTELY a pre-requisite in taking care of other people.

Rick's top tips

1. Use the system and try not to let the system use you.
2. Reach out to others. Find others who support you, with whom you can joke, commiserate or who have your back. Develop a committee of people who are on your side, who can be helpful to you.
3. Establish some kind of personal practice.
4. Find something that disengages and re-centres you and really feeds you from the inside out (e.g. meditation; prayer; reading; art; Pilates; walking the dog or playing music).
5. Take care of your body. Life is a marathon, not a sprint! To sustain a marathon, you have to take care of your body. You have to feed it, give it rest, exercise, pleasure and love. Look for ways to take care of your body and then it will take care of you.

Looking after your own health

CO-FOUNDER OF THE Chiron Centre for Natural Health in Bristol (www.chironcentre.co.uk), which aims at taking complementary health to a new level, Andy Kemp is an inspiring health practitioner who practises what he preaches.

I met Andy when I began training for a half-marathon and had persistent shin pain that would not resolve with normal treatment. He was recommended by a sceptical rugby player who he had cured ... I was interested.

My approach to health has always felt broader than the standard approach that the medical model offers, and my eyes have been opened up to the breadth and depth that health and wellbeing encompass. Andy has helped me and thousands of others in his capacity as a kinesiologist and I continue to learn a huge amount about myself and health from him.

What's the alternative?

There have been fantastic medical advances with the inventions of MRI scans: injection therapy; stem cell treatment, and huge pharmaceutical advances (to mention only a few)... though at what cost?

Do we give our bodies the true respect they deserve by really thinking about what we put into them (whether it be food; drugs or injections) or are we so baffled by science that we forget the power of the body and mind which, when put into operation, are sublime? Does what goes on in our minds, what we feed our bodies, what we watch on TV and what we allow ourselves to be stressed by, affect our bodies? ABSOLUTELY! Should we just neglect the amazing advances in medicine and go for the 'natural' approach? Not necessarily. Modern medicine is powerful, though I think that we have lost touch with the true power inside ourselves that can enhance or complement other forms of treatment.

Conventional medicine has its place. I was trained very conservatively within the medical model approach though I was forced to question it regarding my own health. Understanding my frustrations with the limitations of this conventional medical approach, and allowing myself to be open to the possibilities of the wider world of wellbeing, has taught me so much. As healthcare professionals, we have to allow ourselves to question rather than to blindly conform.

If you are not yet ready to embrace alternative types of healthcare that is OK; I simply ask that you be open to them. You may be surprised by what you learn. After all, your health is surely your most important asset ... why wouldn't you do the best for it, like you would do the best for your patients?

Compassion for your health

We need more compassion, but we forget this when it comes to our own health. When I am ill I feel such a sense of duty towards everyone else that I find it hard to take time off and rest up at home (unless I really can't get out of bed). I know that this is short-sighted and probably prolongs how long I am sick for; I am probably much less effective at all aspects of my job when I am below par. I know I should avoid giving germs to my patients and my colleagues (and would if I was truly unwell). However, I also know that I am not alone. Why can we not have the same compassion for ourselves that we have for everyone else when they are sick?

Ongoing health problems turned out to be Andy's saving grace because they released him from his old patterns. With a seemingly disconnected range of minor symptoms, which generated an ever more disparate range of prescriptions from his GP, he felt at a loss. His life was making him ill, but at the time he had no idea that his emotional balance was key to his physical health. By sheer chance, he overheard a colleague saying how her rheumatism had been helped by a kinesiologist and that a simple detox and change of diet had brought about huge improvements in her symptoms. Intrigued, though sceptical, he made an appointment; his passion developed from this.

For his own wellbeing, Andy has at least two treatments each month (shamanic; kinesiology; massage; shiatsu; cranial sacral and acupuncture). He feels that they add value and help his therapy, which in turn brings more joy and peace into his life.

I was ill when I was writing this, and it made me reflect on how I look after my own health. Prevention is much better than cure – but do we do that with our own health? I have definitely been guilty of taking my health for granted. I push myself, asking a lot from both my mind and body, and get frustrated when I get ill.

Health and wellness happens at a much subtler level than we appreciate and can easily get knocked off balance. When we get symptoms it is often too late. We should learn to be more finely tuned to ourselves and our natural balanced state.

Next time you are sick, stop for a moment before you struggle out of the door, and treat yourself as you would one of your colleagues. Ask yourself if you are well enough to go to work. Be honest and take your own advice.

Taking time to be sensitive to, and learning to listen to, your body is a way to be compassionate. Learning to listen to your gut feelings can be a simple first step.

Gut feeling/intuition

You are probably more than familiar with the feeling of butterflies in your stomach when you think about something that makes you anxious or when you get that *gut feeling* about something that you can't explain logically. Ever been camping and worried about the toilet facilities, only to be relieved that your stomach appears to hold onto its waste products until you get home?! Have you ever stopped to think what causes this and indeed whether you should listen to it?

Recent research has proved that there are nerve cells in your gut that have an awareness and mind of their own! When we have a thought, this is caused by our clever little chemicals, the *neurotransmitters*; we all know these chemical messengers that allow the cells to talk to each other. There are not only receptors to these chemical messengers in our brain cells, but also in other parts of our bodies, for example: *stomach; intestine; colon; kidney*. (In fact, the gut has more nerve cells than the spinal cord.) It has been found that these different parts of the body not only have receptors, but can also make the same chemicals that the brain makes when it thinks. For this reason, some scientists have nicknamed the gut our second brain. So, when you have a *gut feeling* you are probably right!

The gut not only 'thinks' for itself, but is also connected to the part of our brain which controls emotions and behaviour (known as the *limbic system*). A big part of our emotions are influenced by the nerve cells in our gut, so when we are under stress it is often felt in the stomach and intestines first. Butterflies in your stomach is a part of your body's stress response; an upset stomach may be the first sign that you are emotionally upset about something.

So, next time you wonder whether you should trust your instinct and go with your *gut feeling*, maybe you should listen to what it is trying to tell you. The nerve cells in our gut enable us to 'feel' the inner world and are highly connected to our emotions. Becoming more aware of this mind-body link may help you recognise when you are stressed. Every cell in our body responds to every thought and the body can give you clues to this ... all you have to do is listen!

Learn to trust your instincts and how you feel, whether this is in relation to yourself and how you are feeling about something, or in relation to what you feel about a patient.

New challenges

Many healthcare professionals feel that it is becoming more challenging to help their patients. We seem to have deeper issues to address and less capacity to lock them away where they can stew without causing direct symptoms. It is harder now than ever before to be a healthcare practitioner; the reasons for this are multi-faceted:

- The age of accountability
- Transparency of the system
- Patient expectations
- Mistrust of the healthcare systems
- Negative press – focusing on failing hospitals and scandal, with few positive health stories to balance these
- Huge pressure on healthcare practitioners to achieve targets, outputs and objective measures
- A culture of being 'copers'; as healthcare professionals we help everyone else but rarely admit to requiring help ourselves.

Death and injury from medical intervention, secondary infections, the vaccine controversy and waiting lists are all undermining confidence in the NHS. The result of this is paranoia from the health and safety experts, rapidly rising insurance premiums, and overwhelming stress that hangs over us as healthcare professionals. It's no wonder that many of us aren't coping in this current culture!

Historically, healthcare professionals played a supportive role, seeking guidance and inspiration from leaders within the community or from people in positions of power. They aspired to move up the ladder, with success being rewarded by material gain and higher status. Faith in the system helped us make sense of it. For many of us, this faith has been ground away and doesn't exist anymore.

In a wider sense, the media leads us to believe that violence and crime are natural parts of life and that mankind is inherently flawed. This is very damaging to our health, wellbeing and relationships. Personally I don't routinely watch the news as I feel that it is emotionally charged and I have learned that it is not good for my health.

Maybe there is a new way. Andy suggests that it is time for us to stop looking outside for guidance and inspiration, and realise the power we have as individuals. The greatest truths are already within us, waiting to be released. We can't change the system but we can change ourselves and how we work, cope and ultimately thrive within it.

The new paradigm

To help us on this new path, we must believe that true success is available to us all. We need to project what we want to see.

> *'Be the change you want to see in the world.'*
> Mahatma Gandhi

Andy argues that we are in the middle of an exciting global development where we are reclaiming control of our lives, looking for greater fulfilment. We are slowly starting to recognise the futility of a treadmill existence, where we are in huge debt and working forty-five hour weeks to pay it all off. This is no longer enough.

To move onto this new level as individuals, we must leave behind old trauma, illness and fear. Once we find the seed of this inner strength, we start to realise that true healing comes from within. Andy believes that if you search for a wonderful therapist who can take away your pain, you are misguided. The healer is in YOU. All other people can do is show you how to access this inner strength and help you remove the blocks to your own recovery and growth. I think this is very apt for us as healthcare professionals looking deeper into ourselves and healing ourselves, as well as helping our patients.

'Once we start this process, it will evolve continually, expanding beyond our own development to those around us. Just by living and honouring our core values we will influence all those we meet. We all know that kind of person, the one that turns heads when they enter the room, who exudes their truth with every cell in their body and just knows that they are on their optimum path. We must all aspire to be like this.'

If we are prepared to be open and show a little vulnerability in our own health, we find that we are not so different from our colleagues or our patients. We can learn about how our work and the people around us have been affecting us. We can learn to be truly grateful for our own heath. We can make deeper connections with others, whether this is with colleagues or patients. We can learn to do things in a new way and feel what it is like to be truly well and flourish!

Andy's top tips

1. Self-love/care – you must look after yourself to be able to treat patients effectively. As part of this Andy has two treatments a month (consisting of kinesiology, massage, shiatsu, cranial sacral therapy or acupuncture).
2. Daily practice.
3. Interconnectedness – treating others as you wish to be treated.
4. Personality not therapy – the need to be truly engaged in each session with a patient as they are influenced by your energy.
5. Don't look to explore or heal your own issues through your work with others, try to deal with your own stuff separately so you can hold a clean space for your patients.

Practical skills section

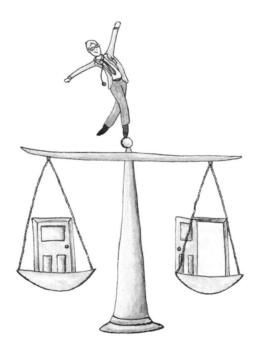

THIS SECTION IS a collection of lots of things that I have learned over the years that I want to share with you … there are lots more that are not covered here.

There is no recipe, and some techniques will work differently or appeal more than others. You need to listen to yourself and what is going on within you; you need to learn to adapt to situations that you find yourself in and sense when you are out of balance. It's like walking a tightrope to try to maintain awareness of how you want to feel each day and what small steps you can take to help you feel that way.

Daily practices

There are lots of subtle shifts that you can choose to do each day that can make a big difference to how you feel or respond to certain situations:

- Setting an intention for the day.
- Gratitude – try recalling five things that you are grateful for from the day just before you go to bed.
- Being present – often we are somewhere else, living in the future. Spend a day where you consciously bring yourself back to the present, really engage with each patient, colleague, loved one... Even at lunchtime, enjoy the present moment of resting and eating.
- Caring/nurturing/rewarding yourself – what small things could you do that care or nurture you? Take the time to make a nutritious breakfast? Take a walk outside at lunchtime? Soak in the bath after work?
- Doing something for fun/pleasure. What do you love to do? Catch up with a friend over coffee or ring a friend for a chat; go dancing or to an exercise class; go to the cinema or watch something that makes you laugh on TV; cook a meal... This list is endless; you just need to get in touch with what gives you pleasure!
- Write yourself a kind/compassionate letter about your day. We are quick to berate ourselves and tell ourselves off for doing what we perceive is a less than perfect job.

What would you say to a friend, colleague or loved one if they told you the things that you are telling yourself?

- Use the act of washing your hands or writing patient notes to say a positive affirmation; repeat a line from a song in your head or be grateful for something.
- Centre and ground yourself in between patients by taking a couple of deep breaths before entering their room or before collecting the next patient from the waiting room. Take a moment to mentally check in with yourself. Notice how you are feeling; are you ready to deal with the next patient?
- Random acts of kindness – compliment a colleague; take some cakes or fruit to work to share; put sticky notes with positive comments on the mirrors in the bathroom or next to the kettle in the staffroom; help another healthcare professional do something you normally wouldn't consider your job; sit and really listen to a patient's story.

'No act of kindness, no matter how small, is ever wasted.'

Aesop

- Employ an 'End of day' practice to help you hang up your professional persona. We put on our professional identities when we begin our working day and some of us forget to step out of them. We need to switch off. What will help you separate from the working day so you can fully engage with your friends, partner or children? It might be the simple act of taking off your uniform and getting changed into your own clothes, locking up your notes, shutting down your computer,

using your commute to listen to some music to switch your state.
- Talk to your partner (or friend or housemate) to offload when you come home from work – they just need to listen for five to ten minutes. No action is required except for active listening – ask for what you NEED!

> *'No matter how much work there is to do… I will find time for pleasure.*
> *No matter how much work there is to do… I will create space for fun.*
> *No matter how much work there is to do… I will have fun!'*

Coping skills

- Reflective writing.
- Stream of consciousness writing. Get a blank piece of paper or a blank computer document and just allow yourself to write. Don't think about what you are writing or censor yourself … allow whatever is inside to flow out.
- Work-life balance.
- What can you practically do to improve the situation? What can you do, together with your colleagues, to help the day go a little better – have a breakfast together, have a break or share things? What could you do to make things better? Go into work and have a meeting where you do this and brainstorm.
- Dealing with emotions: ask a question of your unconscious mind or ask that it gets resolved in your sleep.

- Actively seek to make connections with both colleagues and patients.
- Staff support meetings or 'Schwartz Rounds' – these should involve discussing negative feelings rather than just expecting to cope with them.
- Instead of a boring staff meeting about mundane topics, have a meeting about why you work there; share stories about a beautiful moment with a patient or your own life.
- Read a positive quote or send a positive quote at the beginning of the week; share one at the start of your staff/team meeting.
- Keep your personality – be honest about who you are as a healthcare professional and don't compromise on what feels right to you. Staying true to who you are and showing some of your personality allows for a deeper connection with both patients and other healthcare professionals.

Note to self:

'Treat yourself the way you would treat a small child.
Feed yourself healthy food and make sure you spend time outside.
Put yourself to bed early.
Let yourself take naps.
Don't say mean things to yourself.
Don't put yourself in danger (your skull and your heart are still as fragile as eggshells).'

Physical techniques

- Body scanning
- Yoga
- Breathing techniques
- Meditation: research shows that meditation cultivates empathy by reducing stress, increasing self-compassion and learning to dissociate with one's own subjective perspective (Youngson, 2012, and Neff & Germer, 2012).
- Mindfulness: Dr Dan Siegal has shown that mindfulness can stimulate and strengthen the insular. The stronger and more robust this is, the more empathy you have for others.
- Massage: the skin is linked to the autonomic nervous system and to the immune system. It sends sensory information via touch to the brain and thus can initiate a variety of responses. It is touch which facilitates healing in the tissues.
- Exercise: what keeps you sane? This keeps me sane and I definitely notice the difference when I have had jobs where I can exercise and ones where I can't. What works best for me is to exercise at lunchtimes as it gives me a break in the middle of the day and gets me to switch off. It allows me to refocus on *me* and to refuel with not just food. What does the same for you? How can you work it into your schedule?
- Trauma release exercise: a set of six simple exercises that can assist the body in releasing tension, stress or trauma by evoking muscular shaking (www.bercelifoundation.org).
- Cardiac coherence technique: a quick technique that

can help you balance your emotions, especially when you are starting to feel drained (www.heartmath.org).

Alternate nostril breathing

Close your left nostril with your right ring finger. Inhale for a count of four (through the right nostril only), hold for a count of two before you close the right nostril with your thumb and then exhale for a count of four (through the left nostril only). Repeat for two or three minutes.

Square breathing

Inhaling and exhaling only through your nostrils encourages the 'life force'. Allowing the air to drag over the back of your throat, creating a low, rasping sound as you inhale and exhale is called *Ujjayi* breath. Once you are happy with this breathing technique, you can close your eyes and imagine a square. Inhale along each of the four sides for a count of four, hold for a count of two before exhaling along each of the four sides once again. Repeat for around two to three minutes.

Self-love ritual

Place yourself in a seated, upright position. Begin by focusing on your breath, mentally following the sensation of the air as it flows into your lungs and out again. Feel how your chest rises and falls with each inhale and exhale. Continue this for five to ten minutes.

Next, gently bring into your mind one thing that you don't like about yourself, or one part of yourself that you get frustrated about. Now silently offer that part or that characteristic a blessing of thanks, kindness and love.

Continue to repeat the blessing for the rest of the meditation (maybe another five minutes). Set a timer at the start so you are relaxed about time.

Body awareness exercise

Simply becoming more body aware can be one of the most important tools to help you identify how things (and, in particular, people) affect you and reduce the risk of empathy fatigue. It is something that we are always encouraging our patients to do; it is probably even more important for *ourselves* as the people doing the caring!

Allow yourself to spend ten minutes in a quiet space (where you know you will not be interrupted) and have a go at the following exercise.

Sit comfortably and allow yourself to slowly become aware of your body (closing your eyes may help you focus). Take the time to notice how your skin feels: is it warm or cold? Are there differences in different areas of your body? Notice how your clothes feel next to your skin. Become aware of your feet on the floor and the sensation of your shoes around them.

Next, take some time to notice any areas of tension and areas which feel relaxed. Does one side of your body feel different to the other side?

Now focus your attention to your breathing and just take a few moments to observe it rather than trying to change it. Is it fast or slow, deep or shallow? Do you breathe high up in your chest or low down in your tummy? What about your heartbeat, is it fast or slow?

Moving up to your head and face, notice the expression on your face. Does your mouth and jaw feel relaxed or are they clenched with tension? Take some time to notice how they feel.

Next, allow yourself to remember something or somewhere pleasant from your life (when you felt love, happiness or just a deep sense of relaxation). Notice any changes inside your body and in the areas you have spent time focusing on. Write them down or just take a mental note of them.

Allow yourself to think of something slightly unpleasant or something you are anxious about and note any changes to your body. Return to the pleasant memory to finish with. Open your eyes when you are ready.

Although this is a simple exercise it may take some practice. Allow yourself the time to do it! Practising and noticing how it feels to switch from one memory to another will fine tune your body awareness.

When you feel confident with this exercise you can go on to put it into practice with a patient. Take a few seconds to glance inside your body and take mental note of any feelings you become aware of. Try doing this every twenty minutes or so when you are with a patient. This will also take practice, so be kind to yourself if you forget or if it knocks you off your train of thought!

With practice you will note how you feel when you are interacting with different people and will start to become aware of how some can physically affect you more than others. Also take the time to do this throughout a normal day, noticing anything which causes a change to how you feel inside.

So, have a go and see what you feel from doing this exercise. Allow yourself just to observe what happens inside your body without judging it, even allowing yourself to smile or think "that's interesting" if you notice any changes.

Practical ways to deal with negative emotions

Allowing yourself ways to discharge negative emotion that you may unknowingly absorb from others will really help you. The list below is just a few suggestions:

- Relax and take some deep breaths. Expel any negative emotions with your out breath.
- Writing.
- Removing yourself from the situation.
- Talking to a friend (sometimes just getting it out rather than looking for a solution is all that is needed).
- Offering kindness and positive thoughts to the other person, whether a patient, another healthcare professional or a relative (consciously expressing it to them, if appropriate, or internally expressing it towards them if you don't feel comfortable).
- Washing your hands and imagining the negative energy flowing down the sink and being washed from you/cleansing you.
- Having a shower (e.g. after work to 'wash the negativity off you').
- Imaging yourself surrounded by a protective shield/bubble or a glass bell.
- Imagining the energy flowing between you and the other person and cutting that emotional cord of energy with a pair of scissors.
- Imagine a shower curtain (a clear one) between you and your patient. You can still see and hear everything but this helps you feel there is a soft barrier which is shielding you from their emotions.

- Be present with yourself and check your emotions whilst you sit with a patient. You can listen to a patient whilst mentally checking in with yourself. Recognising how you are feeling and acknowledging that their emotions are not yours.
- Knowing yourself. What do you like? What makes you happy? What drains you? What aspects of your work give you energy? How can you do more of them?

What can you do every day to help develop your own resilience and help you really enjoy each day?

'Seriously, if it is sucking the life out of you, stop giving it your attention. If it's a job you need to quit. If it's a person, cut them out. If it's an activity, by all means, STOP. Stop letting anything but YOU take the wheel. You're going to be okay. Time WILL pass. Get outta there and make your dreams a reality. You don't deserve anxiety. You're not operating at your best when someone or something ELSE is in control. Take over. Get some good vibes cranking and just be happy in your own skin. Love your life. Delete the rest.'

The quiet rabbit

Challenge yourself

How about setting yourself a challenge for the next forty days? Pick one of the practical tools from above, or even better one of your own, and really engage with it. Give it a go and see how it changes you!

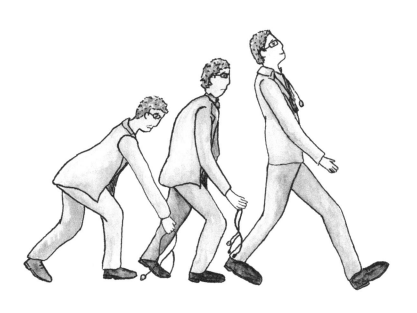

Glossary of terms

Compassion – '*Deep awareness of the suffering of oneself and other living beings, coupled with the wish and effort to alleviate it.*' (Gilbert, 2012).

Empathy – The word empathy comes from the Greek word *Empatheia* which means appreciation of another's feelings. A deep understanding, rather than a feeling. In contrast to sympathy, empathy can be very helpful in your relationship with patients. It can also lead to personal growth, career satisfaction and better clinical outcomes.

Flourishing – to thrive; to live optimally, denoting growth and resilience.

Mindfulness – Intention and non-judgemental focus of attention on emotions, thoughts and sensation.

Reflection – is a '*conscious, active process of focused and structured thinking which is distinct from free-flowing thoughts, as in general thinking or day-dreaming*' (Gelter, 2003).

Resonance – empowers people to design their life in a way that allows them to feel the way they want to feel and about '*getting to the heart of why you as a helper do what you do*' (Newburg et al, 2002).

Self-compassion – the expression of kindness; care and compassion to yourself instead of another.

Sympathy – Largely an emotional attribute that involves intense feelings of another's pain and suffering. It can lead to empathy fatigue, exhaustion and stress. Thus it can be unhelpful for both patient and healthcare professional (Cole-King & Gilbert, 2011, and Youngson, 2012).

Resources

Websites

This is a list of websites that you might find useful.

Compassionate Mind Foundation
(www.compassionatemind.co.uk)

A charity which promotes wellbeing through the scientific understanding and application of compassion. Runs an annual conference in compassion and makes many resources available.

Hearts in Healthcare (www.heartsinhealthcare.com)

A great site founded by Dr Robin Youngson whose aim is to re-humanise healthcare, with articles, inspiration and educational resources.

Kings Fund (www.kingsfund.co.uk)/Schwartz Rounds

An independent charity with the aim of improving healthcare in England through research, development and debate.

Intent.com (www.intent.com)

An online community where you can share your intentions.

The Schwartz Center (www.theschwartzcenter.org)

Set up to honour the legacy of Ken Schwartz in order to nurture compassion in healthcare, this centre supports both patients and their caregivers. The centre runs a range of pioneering educational programmes and events.

Dr Rick Hanson (www.rickhanson.net)

A resource for happiness, love and wisdom.

The Center for Compassion and Altruism Research and Education CCARE (www.ccare.stanford.edu)

This society investigates methods for cultivating compassion within individuals and society through research, education and academic conferences.

Dr Dan Siegle (www.drdansiegle.com)

Home to many resources on how to bring kindness and compassion into work and life from scientific and developmental perspectives. Founder of the 'Mindsight Institute' (www.mindsightinstitute.com) which aims at understanding the mind of the self and others.

The Greater Good Science Centre
(www.greatergood.berkeley.edu)

The centre for the study of psychology, sociology and the neuroscience of well-being, which aims at educating people in skills that develop a thriving, resilient and compassionate society.

Kristen Neff website (www.self-compassion.org)

Run by Dr Kristen Neff, this website provides a wealth of

information about self-compassion for students, researchers and also the general public (including practical exercises and scales for researchers).

Ted.com (www.ted.com)

An inspiring non-profit organisation devoted to spreading ideas across the global community mostly in the form of powerful talks.

Christine Arylo website (www.christinearylo.com)

A positive website all about self-care.

SIRPA website (www.sirpauk.com)

Founded by the pioneering physiotherapist Georgie Oldfield, this site is full of information and resources for both patients and (health)care workers alike.

The Chiron Centre (www.chironcentre.co.uk)

A centre for complementary healthcare co-founded by Andy Kemp.

Doug Newburg (www.dougnewburg.com)

The new website for Doug Newburg with a thought-provoking blog and information on his unique coaching based on 'feel'.

Deepak Chopra website (www.deepakchopra.com)

Incredible visionary who has tirelessly highlighted the mind-body connection in medicine.

Empathy and Compassion in Society
(www.compassioninsociety.org)

Presenting the latest research on how compassion can enhance professional lives, sharing tools for cultivating empathy and compassion as well as case studies.

James Hawkins website (www.goodmedicine.org.uk)

A website by Dr James Hawkins about what makes a 'good life', cutting through a lot of the baffling research out there in the health field.

Kelly McGonigal (http://kellymcgonigal.com)

A health psychologist, lecturer at Stanford University and leading expert in the new field of 'Science-help'. An extensive resource for research on compassion, mindfulness and the effects of emotions.

Compassionate Wellbeing (www.compassionatewellbeing.com)

Hosts events and supports research and activities that promote and explore compassionate approaches to health, wellbeing and society.

Oxford Mindfulness Centre (http://oxfordmindfulness.org)

An international centre of excellence at the forefront of research and development in the field of mindfulness.

Frameworks 4 Change (www.frameworks4change.co.uk)

A great site dedicated to compassion offering training courses, resources, a blog and research studies.

Connecting with People (www.connectingwithpeople.org)

A not-for-profit organisation that develops and delivers training packages, it offers mental health and wellbeing programmes designed to improve support, with particular focus on suicide and self-harm prevention.

Get some headspace (www.getsomeheadspace.com)

A simple resource which aims to help mind health by meditation and offers a free meditation app with some great advice and blog.

Joan Halifax (www.upaya.org)

A Buddhist teacher and pioneer in the field of end-of-life care. She has also spoken and written extensively about gratitude.

www.overexposedthecostofcompassion.weebly.com

A documentary film investigating and explaining 'compassion fatigue'. Produced by MediLab at Pacific Lutheran University, it investigates the lives of professionals whose primary duties are to serve others and the human cost to them.

www.workingwithact.com

A resource that translates the most up-to-date research in behavioural science, mindfulness and Acceptance and Commitment Training (ACT) in the workplace.

www.psychologytools.org

A free resource for therapists to share and develop materials useful to psychological therapists.

www.rachelramen.com

A great resource and blog by the inspirational Rachel Ramen, a clinical professor of family and community medicine at UCSF School of Medicine (one of the pioneers of the Healers' Art – aimed at reintegrating the heart and soul into contemporary medicine to its integrity as a calling and a work of healing).

Heartmath (www.heartmath.com)

A website to help individuals, organisations and the global community incorporate the heart's intelligence into their day-to-day experience of life. Offering products and training to reduce stress, build resilience, and unlock your natural intuitive guidance.

Compassion for Care (www.compassionforcare.com)

The Charter of Compassion for Care is a document that aims to inspire everyone involved to restore compassion as the core principle of healthcare.

Charter for Compassion (www.charterforcompassion.org)

An organisation inspired by the Charter for Compassion that was created by Karen Armstrong. A support to help cultivate cultures of compassion globally through education, business and the arts.

http://www.commonweal.org

A centre for work in healing people and healing the earth set in beautiful Californian countryside. Supports many fields, including programmes in cancer and health professional education.

www.practitionerrenewal.ca

Supporting healthcare practitioners with an aim to enhance well-being, inspire job satisfaction, recharge compassion and mutual support through education and research.

Duke Integrative Medicine
(www.dukeintegrativemedicine.org)

Offering education, professional training and research by using a new approach to medical care. Their approach recognises how the subtle interactions of mind, body, spirit and community interplay and impact on health.

College of Medicine (www.collegeofmedicine.org.uk)

With a vision to inspire, educate and encourage health organisations, practitioners and patients to foster a spirit of equal partnership in health creation and share evidence/experience, and in doing so inspire the health of the future.

www.semel.ucla.edu/cousins/research

The Cousins Centre for Psychoneuroimmunology aims at researching the role of immunological mechanisms that underlie behavioural disturbances with their impacts on mental health.

Awareness in Action (www.awarenessinaction.org)

Awareness in Action offers a view of how to change our working life with the tools to help enable this. With a background in mindfulness, meditation and compassion, Maureen Cooper is the driving force behind this organisation. Offering workshops and online courses, including "compassion in the workplace" in addition to a great blog on reducing stress.

www.theconnection.tv

A feature documentary film revealing the ground-breaking research by world leading experts in mind-body medicine.

Natural Bloom (www.naturalbloom.com)

A great resource for people interested in holistic health worldwide where people can share knowledge with others. Great articles to expand knowledge and a special section on busting stress.

www.workinglives.co.uk

A resource offering advice on how to be more productive, resourceful and happy at work.

Ted Talks (www.tedmed.com)

A health and medicine version of the TED talks (www.ted.com). Talks from inspiring speakers aimed at sharing ideas, discoveries, breakthroughs and passions.

Humans of health.com (www.humansofhealth.com)

An organisation responsible for running the 'Healthcare Leadership Summer School' whose aim is to bring back the true roots of care within healthcare.

www.traumaprevention.com

A resource sharing the tension & trauma release exercise (TRE), a set of exercises aimed at assisting the body in releasing patterns of stress and trauma.

Books

Clarke, D. (2007) *They Can't Find Anything Wrong: 7 Keys to Understanding, Treating and Healing Stress Illness* Sentient Publications. Boulder.

Hanson, R. (2013) *Hardwiring Happiness: The New Brain Science of Contentment; Calm and Confidence Harmony.* New York.

McCourt, J. (2012) *Crushed – My NHS Summer* The University of Buckingham Press. Buckingham.

Newburg, D. (2009) *The Most Important Lesson No One Ever Taught Me* CreateSpace.

Oldfield, G. (2014) *Chronic Pain: Your Key to Recovery* AuthorHouse UK. London

Richardson, C. (2009) *The Art of Extreme Self-care* Hay House UK. London.

Rothschild, B. (2006) *Help for the Helper: The Psychophysiology of Compassion Fatigue and Vicarious Trauma* W.W. Norton and Company. New York.

Sapolsky, R. (2004) *Why Zebras Don't Get Ulcers* St Martins Press. New York.

Sarno, J. (2008) *The Divided Mind: The Epidemic of Mindbody Disorders* Gerald Duckworth & Co Ltd. London.

Turnbull, G. (2012) *Trauma: From Lockerbie to 7/7: How trauma affects our minds and how we fight back* Corgi. London.

Youngson, R. (2012) *Time to Care: How to love your patients and your job* RebelHeart Publishers. Raglan, New Zealand.

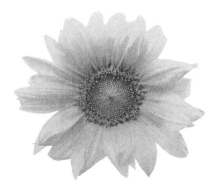

Lightning Source UK Ltd.
Milton Keynes UK
UKOW06f1329270715

255880UK00013B/285/P